The Running School
for Kids

A children's guide to better, faster running technique!

This book belongs to

_____

Before we begin, please make a note of what you'd like to achieve with running or sport and what you'd like to improve. For instance, I wanted to improve my speed and acceleration so I could make the first team in football at school!

Things I'd like to improve in my running:

_____

_____

_____

_____

Things I'd like to achieve in running or sport:

_____

_____

_____

_____

We'll review your progress at the end of the book!

Contents

Welcome to The Running School!

Welcome to The Running School, where YOU get to become the best runner you can be!

Running isn't just about putting one foot in front of the other—it's a skill, just like riding a bike or playing a game. And guess what? Anyone can learn to do it better—even you!

Maybe you love running and want to get faster, or maybe you're not a fan of running yet, and that's okay too. By the time you finish this book, you'll know how to run with confidence, skill and most importantly with great running technique!

In this book, I'll teach you all the cool things about running: a little bit of history, how your body works, what good running technique looks like and what common running mistakes to avoid, and even some tricks to make you faster.

Don't worry—this isn't about running the fastest race or being perfect. It's about learning, having fun, and seeing what your body can do.

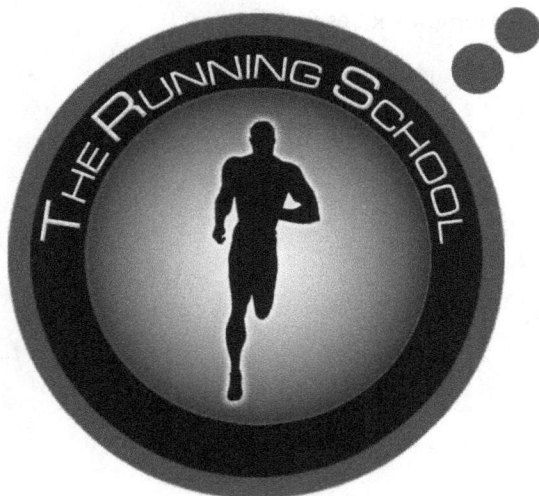

Your Running Technique Coach

I'm Nick, and I'm excited to be your coach in this book. I've been a coach at The Running School and teaching kids and adults how to run since 2010. I've taught everyone from 5 year olds to Premier League footballers and Olympians and let me tell you—everyone can improve their running!

The Running School was started by my Dad, Mike Antoniades. I've been lucky enough to be a part of his team for over a decade and I can now say that I have a pretty good running technique but that wasn't always true. As a kid I was always very active, playing football and Taekwondo from a young age so you'd think I'd have a good running style what with my Dad being a movement Guru and all!

When I was old enough to go to the first Running School in London to have my running analysed, Mike said that I have a very 'unique' running technique, which I now know means I needed a lot of work! It didn't take long to improve my running and The Running School has developed a unique way of coaching kids and adults how to run better in a short space of time, all it takes is some practice.

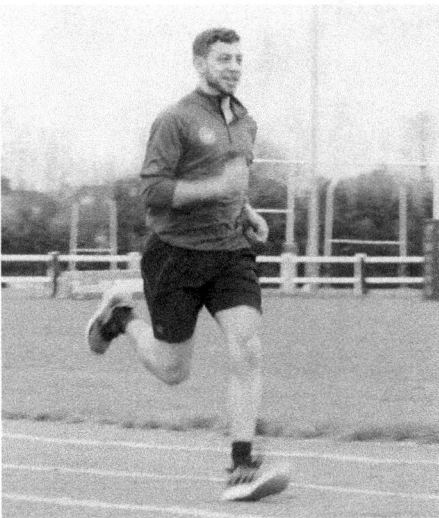

Me practising my running technique!

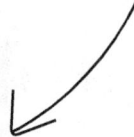

Each day at The Running School is different, we work with everyone from people who have been told they'd never run again to Olympic gold medalists. I get to see runners like you discover how amazing running can be, and nothing makes us happier than watching kids find their confidence on the running track, on the football pitch, or even just in their local parkrun.

Over the years, I've learned a lot about running, and now I get to help you learn how to run better, faster and for longer! In this book, I'm going to share everything I've taught to hundreds if not thousands of young runners.

Your running technique coach and biggest fan,

Nick

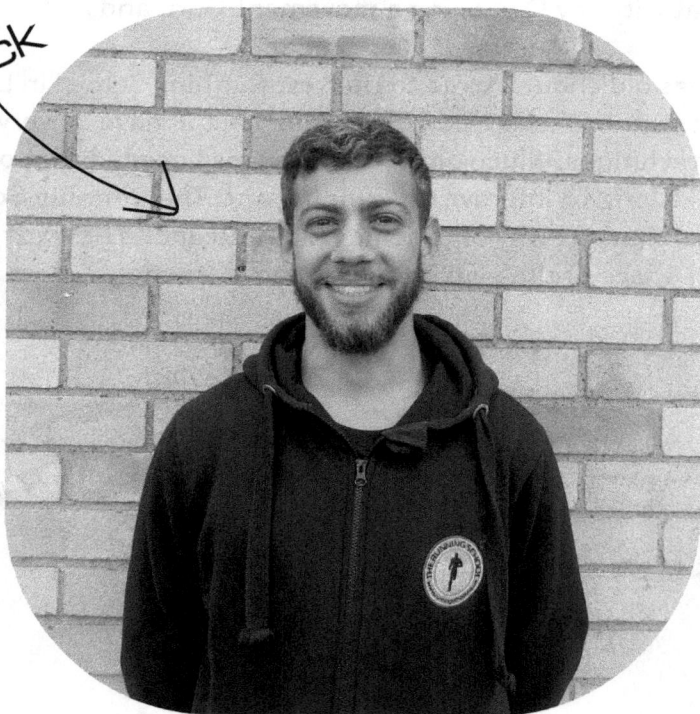

Nick

The Running School

Our Philosophy

At The Running School, we believe that to run faster, you first need to move better! We've spent over 30 years helping people get better at moving, whether they're athletes, beginners, or even those who've had injuries.

The Running School was founded in 1994 by Mike Antoniades, more on him later. Since then The Running School has gone on to coach thousands of people around the World helping them to **Move Better, Run Better and Run Faster**. The Running School now has 40 partner locations and certified coaches worldwide from London to Europe, Asia, North America and more.

We help:
- People who aren't athletes, those who've had injuries or surgery, and kids who need help with their movement.
- Kids as young as 6 years old by teaching them how to move their bodies well and run better.
- Everyone, from beginner runners to experienced runners, and professional athletes from football, rugby, basketball, handball, track and field, and more. We've even worked with Olympians and World Champions!
- We also work with national rugby, football teams and Olympic teams from different countries, helping their coaches and staff learn how to train better.

Our special techniques for teaching running and improving movement have helped us work with kids, beginners and professional athletes for over 30 years.

Learning to run is like learning a new musical instrument or language, you'll only get better with practice. So be sure to practice your homework each week and you'll be running better in no time!

WHY RUNNING IS AWESOME!

Why Running is Awesome!

Running is, in my opinion, the easiest sport to be a part of. You don't need fancy equipment or expensive clothes or trainers—just you, your shoes, and the open space around you. Here are some cool reasons why running is great:

Running is one of the best ways for kids to stay active, have fun, and build a strong, healthy body. It's something anyone can do—whether you're racing friends, playing a sport, or just running around the playground. Here's why running is so important for children:

It Makes You Stronger & Faster
Running helps build strong muscles and bones, which is super important as kids grow. It improves speed and endurance, so you can run longer without getting tired. It teaches better coordination and balance, which helps with all sports and activities.

It's Great for Your Heart & Lungs
Running keeps your heart healthy by making it stronger. It improves how well your lungs work, helping you breathe easier when playing sports. The more you run, the more energy you'll have for other activities.

It Helps You Feel Happier & Less Stressed
Running releases happy chemicals (endorphins) that boost your mood. It helps reduce stress and anxiety, so you feel calmer and more focused. Running outside in nature can help you feel more relaxed and refreshed.

It Helps You Sleep Better
Running burns off extra energy, making it easier to fall asleep at night. Kids who run and play during the day sleep longer and deeper, which helps them feel great the next morning!

It's Fun & Easy to Do!
You don't need fancy equipment—just a pair of shoes and a place to run! You can run anywhere—in the park, at school, or even in your backyard. It's fun to challenge yourself to run faster or longer each time!

It Helps in Other Sports
Whether you play football, basketball, gymnastics, or rugby, running makes you faster, stronger, and more agile. It helps improve your reaction time and coordination, making you better at all kinds of movement.

It Keeps You Healthy & Prevents Injuries
Running boosts your immune system, which helps your body fight off colds and illnesses. It makes your muscles and joints stronger, reducing the chances of getting hurt in other activities.

So, whether you run to play, to stay healthy, or just because it feels good, running is one of the simplest and coolest things you can do.

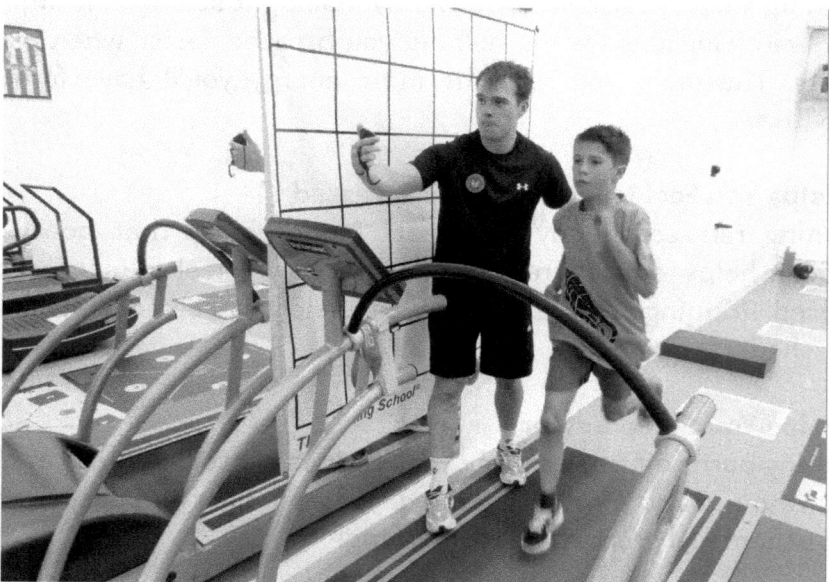

THE HISTORY OF RUNNING

The History of Running: From Cavemen to Champions

Human beings have been running for millions of years. Running isn't just something we do for fun or sport—it's something we've done to survive, explore, and even change the world! Here are some amazing moments from the history of running:

Why Did Humans Start Running?
Did you know that humans have been running for millions of years? Running didn't start as a sport—it was something early humans needed to do to survive!

How Running Began
A long time ago, our ancient ancestors, called Australopithecus, were some of the first creatures to walk on two legs. Scientists believe that around 2.6 million years ago, humans became endurance runners—meaning they could run for long distances.

One way early humans used running was for persistence hunting—this means they would chase an animal until it got too tired to run away. Over time, the human body developed special features to make running easier, like:

• Strong Achilles tendons (helping us push off the ground)
• Big knee joints (absorbing impact)
• Muscular glutes (bum muscles) (giving us power to run)
• Sweat glands (keeping us cool so we could run longer)

Because of these changes, humans became some of the best long-distance runners in the animal kingdom!

The First Marathon

Have you ever heard of a "marathon"? It's a race that's 26.2 miles long —that's a LOT of running! But did you know the marathon started as a real-life story from ancient Greece?

A long time ago, in 490 BC, a soldier named Pheidippides ran all the way from a town called Marathon to Athens to deliver an important message. The Greek army had just won a big battle, and he ran 25 miles to tell everyone about it. He shouted, "We Win!" and then, according to legend, collapsed because he was so tired.

Today, people all over the world run marathons to challenge themselves and honour Pheidippides' incredible run.

Running in Ancient Times

Running wasn't just for hunting or delivering messages—it became a sport too! In ancient Greece, runners competed in the Olympics, which started over 2,700 years ago. One of the most popular events was a race called the "stadion," which was about 200 meters long. Back then, athletes didn't even wear shoes—they ran barefoot!

Modern Running Races

Fast forward to the 1800s and 1900s, and running became a big part of sports competitions. The first modern Olympics in 1896 included running races, and marathon running became one of the most exciting events. Over time, runners from all over the world started breaking records, running faster, and inspiring others to lace up their shoes.

Famous Moments in Running

Roger Bannister's Mile: In 1954, a man named Roger Bannister became the first person to run a mile in under 4 minutes. People thought it was impossible, but he proved them wrong! The remarkable thing is, however, that one month later another runner also ran under 4 minutes. In the following year, more and more people started to break the 4-minute mile. When you believe you can achieve!

Kipchoge's Amazing Run: In 2019, Eliud Kipchoge from Kenya became the first person to run a marathon in under 2 hours!

A Running School Runner Breaks The World Record: Susannah Gill *(below)* is a British runner who became famous for an incredible challenge called the World Marathon Challenge. In 2019, she ran seven marathons on seven continents in seven days—and she did it faster than anyone before! Her total running time was 24 hours, 19 minutes, and 9 seconds, beating the old record by more than three hours! She ran in Antarctica, South Africa, Australia, the United Arab Emirates, Spain, Chile, and the United States. Susannah even wrote a book with the Founder of The Running School, Mike Antoniades, called "Running Around the World: How I Ran 7 Marathons on 7 Continents in 7 Days", where she shares how she trained with The Running School and what the experience of that amazing race was like.

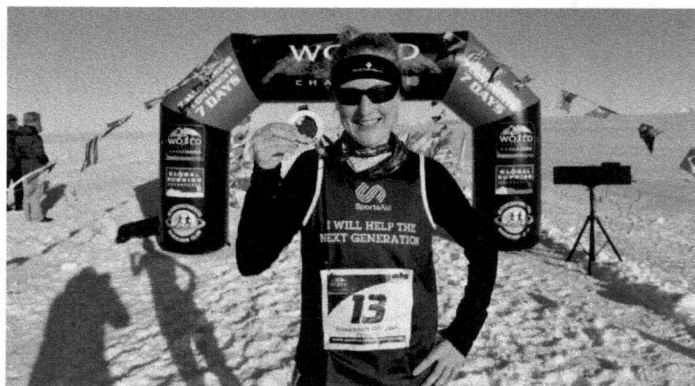

Famous Runners Who Started Just Like You

Even the world's greatest runners had to start somewhere! Here are a few inspiring runners you should know about:

Eliud Kipchoge – Eliud is one of the fastest marathon runners in history. In 2019, he became the first person to run a marathon in under 2 hours! He says, *"No human is limited,"* which means with practice, you can do amazing things too.

Usain Bolt – Known as the fastest man on Earth, Usain Bolt holds the world record for the 100-meter sprint, running it in just 9.58 seconds! When he was younger, he didn't take running seriously preferring football and basketball, but with the right training, he became a legend.

Mo Farah – Mo Farah is a British long-distance runner who won Olympic gold medals for both the 5,000 meters and 10,000 meters. Even when he was the best in the World, Mo still did multiple running technique practice sessions a week.

Paula Radcliffe – Paula is one of the greatest female marathon runners in history. She set the women's marathon world record in 2003 and held it for an incredible 16 years! When she was a child, she loved running because it made her feel strong and free. Paula shows us that hard work, determination, and a love for running can lead to record-breaking success.

These runners prove that no matter where you start, you can become a better runner with practice, belief in yourself, and the right mindset. Who knows? One day, you might be the one inspiring others to run!

RUNNING
IS A
SKILL

Why Running is a Skill You Can Improve

What Is a Skill?

A skill is something you learn to do through practice and effort. It's not something you're just born with—it's something you get better at the more you do it! For example: Tying your shoelaces or riding a bike – At first, it was tricky, but with practice, you got better.

Even though most people can run, running well is a skill. With the right technique, you can run faster, for longer, and with less effort—just like learning how to kick a ball properly in football or do a perfect cartwheel in gymnastics (I've personally given up on this one).

The best part? Skills can always be improved! The more you practice, the better you get. So if you want to become a great runner, keep practicing, and soon, it will feel easy and natural!

Here's a sneak peek at the awesome things you'll discover in this book:

How to run with great technique: Did you know there's a "right" way to run? You'll learn how to move your feet, arms, and body so running feels easier and faster.

How to improve your running technique: With fun homework sessions and tips, you'll be able to run better and feel great while doing it.

How to avoid common running mistakes: We'll show you the common mistakes runners make and how to correct them.

How to improve your speed, balance & coordination: With some more fun (but tough) drills, I'll show you how to improve your speed for sport, and your balance and help improve the connection between your brain and feet that controls coordination.

Why is Running Technique Important?

Why Is Running Technique Important for Children?
Running is something most kids do naturally, but did you know that learning the right technique can make running easier, faster, and more fun? Having good running form helps children move more efficiently, avoid injuries, and build confidence in sports and everyday activities. Here's why I think running technique matters:

It Helps You Run Faster
Good technique means your body moves smoothly without wasting energy. When you use the right arm drive, posture, and leg movement, you can run faster with less effort.

It Prevents Injuries
Poor running form—like overstriding, stomping, or twisting—can put stress on your knees, ankles, and hips. Learning to land lightly and use the right muscles protects your joints and keeps you running without pain.

It Saves Energy
Running with the wrong technique can tire you out quickly because your body is working harder than it needs to. Good form helps you run longer without feeling exhausted.

It Improves Balance & Coordination
When you run with the right technique, your body stays stable and balanced. This helps in other sports too—whether you're playing football, basketball, rugby, or gymnastics.

It Builds Confidence & Makes Running Fun!
When running feels easy and natural, you'll enjoy it more and want to keep doing it. Feeling strong and fast can boost self-confidence in races, sports, and everyday play.

Kids vs. Adults

Why Kids and Adults Train Differently
Your body is different from an adult's body, and so is the way you grow and get stronger. For this reason, we need to coach you differently to how we'd coach an adult. There are certain things you shouldn't do until you're older, such as heavy weights, as this may cause injuries.

Kids Are Still Growing
Your bones, muscles, and joints are growing all the time. That's why it's super important to be careful and not push too hard when you're running. Adults are already fully grown, so their training is more about keeping their bodies strong and healthy. For you, running should be about having fun and learning step by step.

Kids Have More Energy (and Love to Play!)
If you've ever noticed that adults get tired faster than you when you're playing or running around, it's because kids naturally have more energy for short bursts of activity. You learn best by playing games, trying fun challenges, and mixing up your runs with lots of variety.

Kids Learn Faster
Your brain is amazing at learning new skills, like running with good technique! Adults can learn too, but it usually takes them a little longer to pick up new movements. That's why now is the perfect time to practice your running skills—it's easier to learn when you're younger!

Rest Is Important
Because you're still growing, your body needs lots of rest. That's how your muscles, bones, and energy get stronger. Adults need rest too, but for kids, it's extra important. After all, you're busy running, jumping, climbing, and doing a hundred other things every day!

What This Means for You
You don't need to train like an adult to get better at running. You'll improve by practising good technique, staying active, and most importantly, having fun. Running should never feel like a chore—it's something you do to feel strong, fast, and happy.

So remember: kids aren't mini-adults. Your training should be playful, exciting, and designed just for you. And guess what? That's exactly what this book is here to help you with!

THE
FUNDAMENTALS OF RUNNING TECHNIQUE

Why Kids Run the Way They Do

When you're between 6 and 10 years old, your body is still figuring out how to move the best way it can—kind of like learning to play a new video game or musical instrument. Even if you're very active or playing lots of sports, you might not have full control over your movements yet.

Here's what that looks like:
- You might take quick, noisy steps when you run, stomping hard on the ground.
- Your arms might not know what to do, so they don't help as much as they should.

When you try to run faster, you might:
- Take big, long steps that make you lean too far forward (and maybe feel like you're going to tip over!).
- You might tilt your head back too far or swing your arms across your body.

Sometimes, when kids watch their parents or athletes on TV, they try to copy their moves—but it doesn't always look quite the same. That's because your body is still learning how to work together, and sometimes your arms and legs don't quite agree yet.

But here's the awesome part: Kids are amazing at learning! Your brain can adapt and get better really quickly. At The Running School, we've seen kids go from wobbly and noisy runners to smooth and strong ones in just one hour of practice.

With the right tips and a little practice, your running can improve faster than you think.

There's No Such Thing as the Perfect Runner!

Did you know there's no perfect way to run? That's right! But there is a way that's perfect for *you*. Why? Because everyone's body is a little different. Some of us are tall, some are short, some are super flexible, and others are still building strength.

For example:

The fastest way to land when you run is usually on the ball of your foot (the part just behind your toes). Landing like this helps you:

* Stay light on your feet, so you spend less time on the ground.
* Avoid injuries because you don't hit the ground as hard.
* Run faster and use less energy.

But here's the thing: not everyone can run this way. Some people might land differently because their body isn't strong enough, they've had an injury, or they're just used to doing it another way. Even some world-class runners don't always land on the balls of their feet!

At The Running School, we try to teach every child how to land on the balls of the feet, so you can have that skill in your locker to use it when you need to. For adults, it can take up to a year to change the way they land!

We're going to teach you the correct way to run and then we'll have to practice until it becomes *your* perfect technique!

What Does Great Running Look Like?

Changing your running technique is simple, but it's not easy. It'll take a few weeks of practice until it feels comfortable but by the end running should feel easy, light and steady.

Your arms? They should swing back and forth, relaxed but powerful, like little pistons in a machine. And your legs? They should move like they're cycling—when your foot comes off the ground, your heel lifts toward your bottom. This helps you move fast and smoothly!

In this next section, we're going to break down what great running technique should look like.

Let's start from the ground up.

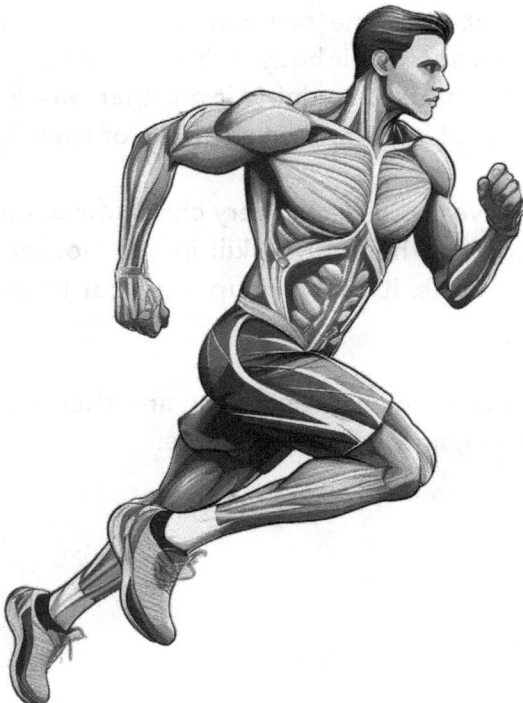

RUNNING
TECHNIQUE

Feet

Where Should Your Feet Land?

When you run, your feet should land just ahead of your centre of gravity, not way out in front of you. Imagine your body has an invisible line running straight down from your belly button to the ground—your feet should touch down just ahead of that line.

Why is this important? Well, if your feet land too far in front of you, it's called "over-striding," and it's like putting on the brakes every time you take a step. You slow yourself down, and running feels harder than it needs to.

It's by far the most common thing we have to fix here at The Running School. Mainly because most of us naturally think that to run faster you have a take a longer step, well that's not true. All the power comes from us pushing off the ground behind us.

Think of a Wheel vs. a Braking Car

Imagine a smooth, rolling bicycle wheel. It moves forward without stopping or slowing down. That's what good running feels like when your feet land underneath you!

Now picture a car hitting its brakes—every time your foot lands way out in front, it's like the car stop suddenly. It takes extra effort to get moving again, and it doesn't feel very smooth, does it?

Okay, now how should your feet land?

Landing

Heel-Toe

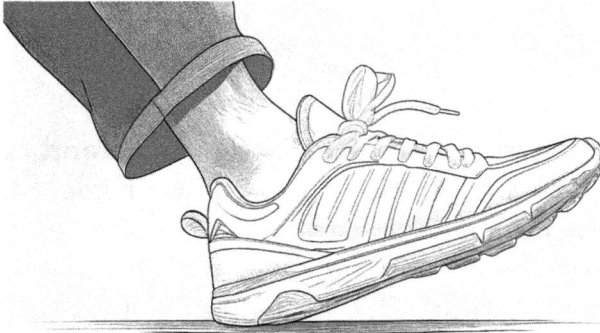

Mid-foot

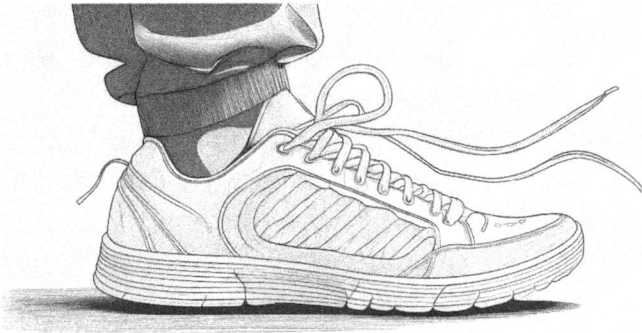

Fore-foot

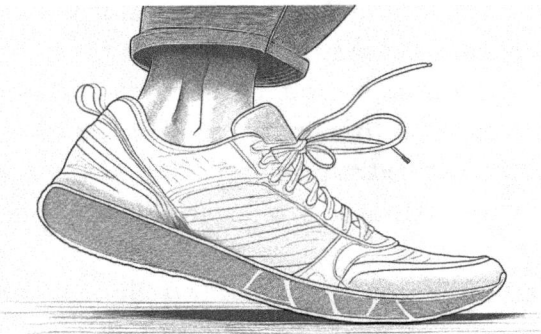

How Should Your Feet Land?

When we run, there are three ways your foot can hit the ground. Heel-Toe, Mid-foot and Fore-foot. All three have their benefits and there's no right or wrong way it depends on you as the runner and what speed you're running.

Heel-Toe

This is how most runners land. It feels comfortable and natural because that's how we walk. When you walk, your heel touches the ground first. For me, landing Heel-toe is best for my slower runs, saving energy and running over rough terrain like cross-country runs. Sometimes I'll change back to heel-toe when I'm tired.

Mid-foot

Landing on your midfoot means the middle part of your foot (just behind your toes) touches the ground first.

Your foot lands softly and evenly, almost flat, so the middle of your foot and heel touch the ground at nearly the same time. It's light and easy on your body. Your knees, hips, and back don't get as much stress because the landing is gentle. It's great for everyday running or long distances. Landing mid-foot can be hard to master.

Fore-foot

Landing on your forefoot means the front part of your foot (the ball of your foot, near your toes) hits the ground first.

Your heel stays off the ground, so you feel springy and bouncy, like a football player or a sprinter. It's great for running fast! Landing on the forefoot gives you an extra push forward, almost like you're on springs. Sprinters and athletes often use this for speed.

It's important that you know how to land depending on the situation and you've got the skills to pick and choose when you use it.

Leg Cycle

What's The Biggest Muscle in Your Body?
I'll give you a clue...you sit on it all day at school!

That's right! The muscle in your bum is the largest in the human body. It's called the gluteus maximus or can otherwise be known as the glutes.

Your bum muscles are one of the most important muscles in our body when it comes to walking and running. The problem is that we sit down too much; at school, at home, and in the car. We need to get these power muscles working!

When I'm coaching people at The Running School, one of the most common issues is that they're not using their glutes enough and this becomes more of a problem when you're older and start driving everywhere, working in an office and sitting around in meetings.

Where Should Your Legs Move?
When your foot comes off the ground, the back of your foot (your heel) should lift up toward your bum—almost like you're kicking yourself in the backside! *(Don't actually kick yourself, but almost!)*. There's a difference between butt flicks and a leg cycle.

Why do this? It makes the muscles in the back of your leg (called your hamstrings) and your bum (your gluteus maximus) work together, helping you run stronger.

This movement creates a smooth, cycling motion, like pedalling a bike. It also helps you land in the correct position and reduce your over-stride, more on that later.

Changing the way your legs move can be the hardest of all the running technique changes we're going to introduce.

You may find that lifting your heels higher is more tiring, and it should be! You'll be using new muscle groups in your glutes and hamstrings and you'll also need a lot more brain power to focus on running with good technique!

It may also feel very strange but with enough practice, it'll get much easier.

It may take anything from two weeks to eight weeks until your leg cycle starts to feel more comfortable. As one of our Running School coaches Joe used to say 'It's not practice makes perfect' but 'perfect practice makes permanent'.

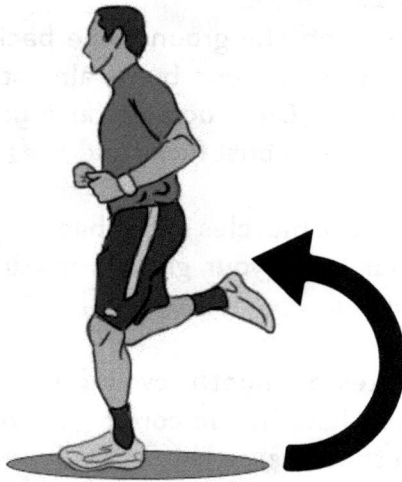

Arm Drive

How to Use Your Arms When You Run
Your arms and legs work together like a team when you run! If your arms move the right way, they help keep your body smooth and steady. Your arms should be thought of as an engine, the faster your arms move the faster your legs will go!

Sweets in Your Pockets!
Imagine your hand is a little rocket travelling from your hip to your chin. Swing your arm backwards toward your hip and then forward to the chin or shoulder level. This keeps your arms moving in the right path—smooth and powerful! At The Running School, I tell everyone to imagine you've got sweets in your jacket pockets, take a sweet and pop it in your mouth *(don't use real sweets!)*

Hands
The hand should be in a light fist as if holding a butterfly or an egg. Don't squeeze too tight, or you'll break the egg! If your hands are too relaxed and floppy then the muscles in your arm will switch off, we need all our muscles working together.

Elbows Bent
Keep your elbows bent at a right angle, like the letter "L," between 45 and 90 degrees. Don't let them go floppy or too straight.

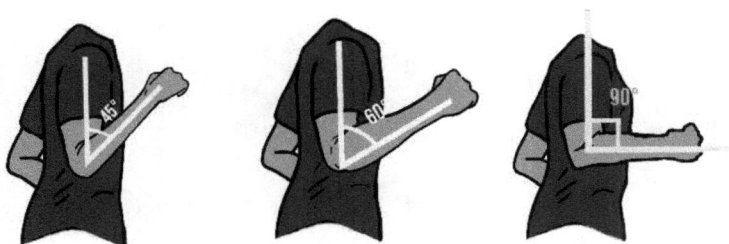

Drive Elbows Back
Focus on pushing your elbows backward rather than swinging your hands forward. It might feel strange at first, but it keeps your motion strong and helps your legs move better, too. Imagine you're pulling on invisible strings behind you!

Relax Shoulders
Don't let your shoulders scrunch up toward your ears—keep them relaxed and loose. This helps you run smoothly without any extra tension.

Posture

Keep Tall

How you hold your body when you run—your posture—makes a big difference! Good posture helps you run faster, reduces your over-stride, and helps reduce your risk of knee or back injuries. Let's learn how to stand tall like a champion!

Stand Tall

Imagine a balloon gently pulling you up from the top of your head. Keep your back straight and your chest slightly lifted.

Keep Your Chin Level

Look ahead, not down at your feet. Imagine you're spotting a finish line or a friend waving at you from far away. This keeps your neck relaxed and your body in line.

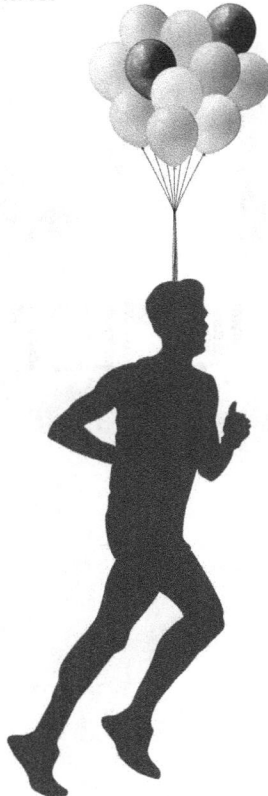

COMMON MISTAKES AND INEFFICIENCIES

How to Analyse Your Own Running Technique

Before you start, video yourself running. Get a friend or family member to take a video of your current running technique. One from the side and one each from the back and front. You can use your phone or a camera for this. If you're able to film in slow motion or slow the video down after then that's even better. It's easy to miss things with fast runners!

Take the same videos again and compare your running before and after you complete the Running Technique Homework plan at the end of the book. This will help you to see your progress after you have finished the full programme.

In this next section we're going to take a look at the most common ineficiencies I see with kids I work with at The Running School.

You may find that you're doing some of these things when you run or just one or two.

Excessive Overstride

What is Overstriding?
Overstriding is when you stretch your leg out too far in front of you while running. It's one of the most common mistakes runners make.

When you overstride, your foot lands way ahead of your hips, which is not the best way to run. Your foot should land just a little bit in front of your body.

Why is Overstriding a Problem?

It Hurts Your Body
When your foot lands too far ahead, your leg has to take on extra weight. This can put stress on your ankles, shins, knees, hips, and even your back.

It Slows You Down
Imagine running downhill and needing to stop—you stick your feet out in front to brake, right? Overstriding is like pressing the brakes, even on flat ground. This makes you slower.

Too Much Ground Time
Overstriding means your foot hits the ground sooner and stays there longer. The longer your foot stays on the ground, the harder it is to stay fast and avoid injuries.

Common Myth
Many people believe that if you land on your heel you are automatically overstriding and that if you're landing forefoot, it stops you from over-striding.
The truth is, you can overstride no matter how your foot lands. Even runners who land on their forefoot can overstride if their foot is too far in front of their body. On the flip side, it's also possible to run well and not overstride, even if you land on your heel. What really matters is where your foot lands in relation to your body.

Using the Wrong Muscles

When you overstride, you rely too much on the muscles at the front of your legs (your quads and hip flexors). These muscles are smaller and not as powerful as the muscles at the back of your legs (your glutes and hamstrings). Your glutes and hamstrings are like rockets—they're what make you faster and stronger!

Harder to Go Fast

Overstriding makes running feel harder. It's tough to pick up speed because you're not using your "power muscles" (glutes and hamstrings) as much as you can.

Bad Posture

Overstriding can make you lean forward too much at your hips. When you lean like this, it's harder to use your back leg muscles properly, making running less powerful.

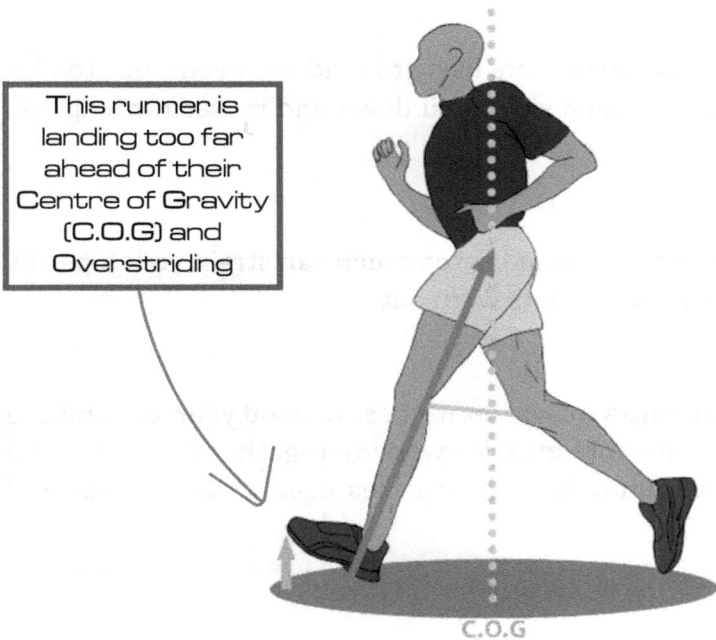

This runner is landing too far ahead of their Centre of Gravity (C.O.G) and Overstriding

C.O.G

Low Heel Lift

What is Low Heel Lift?

When you run, your heel should lift up toward your bum after it leaves the ground. But with some runners, it doesn't lift high enough. Low heel lift means your heel is coming up lower than your knee like you're keeping your leg almost straight.

This happens because the muscles at the front of your leg (like your quads and hip flexors) are doing most of the work to swing your leg forward. It's like trying to run with a long stick instead of a springy leg!

Why is Low Heel Lift a Problem?

Tired Legs

When you run like this, your quads (the muscles at the front of your thighs) get tired quickly. This makes long runs or sprints harder.

Overstriding

A straight leg means you're more likely to land with your foot too far in front of your body, which slows you down and makes running less efficient.

Hip Pain

Using the front muscles of your leg too much can strain your hips. It's like overusing a tool until it gets worn out.

Not Very Efficient

When you try to pick up a heavy box it's best to bend your legs and use both arms to lift, the more muscles working together the better. We want the same for running, more muscles equals more power and better efficiency.

How to Fix It

Lift That Heel!
Try bringing your heel up higher—like you're kicking yourself in the bum. This helps bend your knee more and makes your running smoother.

Use Your "Power Muscles"
Focus on using the big muscles at the back of your legs (your glutes and hamstrings) to swing your leg forward instead of relying only on the front muscles.

Why It's Worth It
When you lift your heel higher, running feels lighter, and faster, and eventually, it'll feel much easier. Plus, it's easier on your joints and muscles, so you can reduce your risk of injuries as you get older!

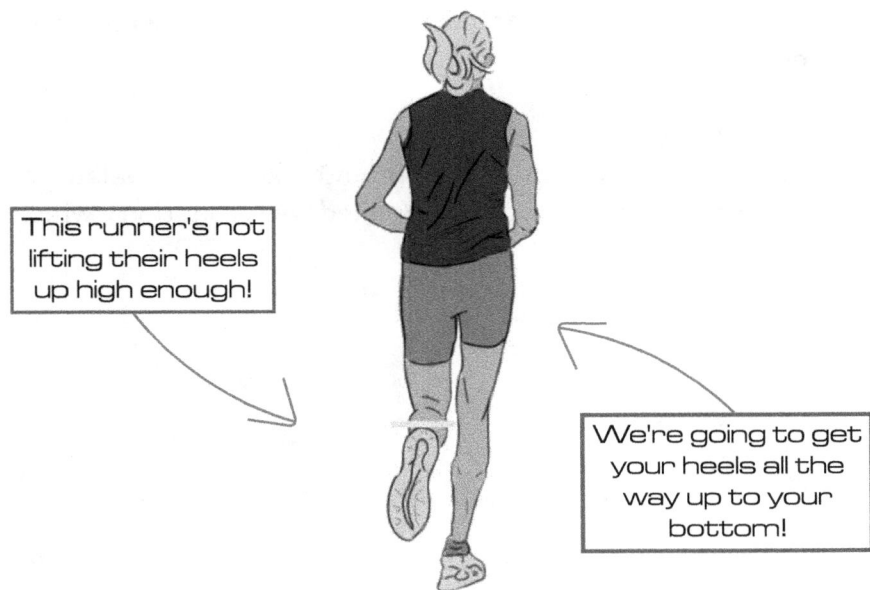

This runner's not lifting their heels up high enough!

We're going to get your heels all the way up to your bottom!

Cross Over

What is Cross-Over?
Cross-over happens when your foot lands too close to the middle of your body like you're walking on a tightrope instead of on train tracks. This can throw your body out of balance and put extra pressure on parts like your knees, ankles, hips, and back.

Why is it a Problem?
When your feet cross over, the joints in your ankles, knees and hips don't line up the way they should. This can lead to:

Knee Pain
Your knees take on extra pressure when your steps aren't aligned. This can also strain something called the IT band (a stretchy band that runs along the outside of your leg).

Hip Pain
If your IT band is working too hard, it can cause pain in your hip or along the outside of your thigh.

Ankle and Foot Pain
Your ankles and feet have to work harder to keep you balanced. Sometimes, your foot rolls in too much (called overpronation), which can cause problems.

Achilles Pain

The Achilles tendon (a strong band at the back of your ankle) can get stressed when your feet and ankles are trying to make up for poor alignment.

Back Pain

If the lower part of your body isn't moving right, your back might twist or tilt to compensate, which can make it ache.

How to Fix It

To stop cross-over, we need to improve your single-leg strength and balance, the single-leg jumps in our Dynamic Movement Skills section will help you to do this! Don't try and run with your feet wider apart as you'll end up looking like a cowboy trying to run after a long horse ride!!

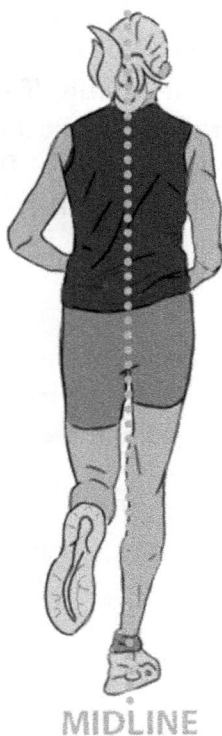

> See how this runner is landing with one foot too close to their midline.

MIDLINE

Inefficient Arm Movement

Why Are Arms Important When Running?

Your arms aren't just there to swing around when you run—they play a very important role! They help you:

- Run faster
- Stay balanced
- Keep a steady rhythm

But did you know that how you move your arms can also affect how your legs work? If your arms are doing something funny, like swinging too much or crossing in front of your body, it can throw off your whole run.

What Happens If You Don't Use Your Arms Properly?

Not Using Your Arms Enough

Our bodies need rhythm when we run. If you don't swing your arms much, your body has to work harder in other ways—like twisting your upper body, which can waste energy. Plus, swinging your arms backwards helps push your body forward, so it's really important to do this!

Crossing Over Your Body

If your arms cross in front of you like an X, it can make your upper body twist too much or mess up your legs by causing them to cross over. This actually slows you down and can lead to injuries as you get older.

Swinging Elbows Too Much

Your elbows shouldn't bend and straighten like crazy while you run. Keep your elbows bent at a nice, steady angle to save energy. This is especially true if you're running long distances.

Straight Arms (Long Lever)

If your arms are too straight, they become like long levers, which are harder to swing and slow you down. It's also connected to running with straight legs, which isn't very efficient.

How Should You Use Your Arms When Running?

- Bend your elbows at about 45-90 degrees (like making an L-shape with your arm).
- Focus on driving your arms backwards, not just forward. This helps you move faster!
- Keep your hands relaxed (like you're holding an egg) and swing your arms forward and backwards, not across your body.

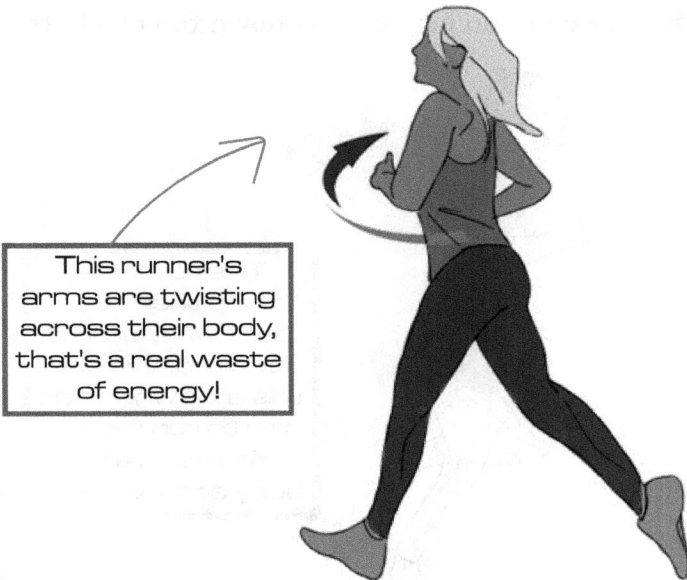

This runner's arms are twisting across their body, that's a real waste of energy!

Head Posture

One thing we must not forget to mention is head posture. The whole body is involved in running – including our head.

If your head is in the wrong position, it can mess with your posture and the way your body moves. Sometimes, poor head position happens because your posture isn't right. Other times, your head might tilt or lean because something lower in your body is out of alignment.

What Happens If Your Head Is in the Wrong Position?
Imagine if you're leaning forward too much from your hips. To see where you're going, your neck has to tilt back so your head stays level. This might feel normal, but it can actually put a lot of strain on your neck and shoulders.

If you look down too much when you run, you'll start to lean forwards which can lead to over-striding and that slows you down.

I see a lot of kids lift their chin too high or look down too much, try and keep your chin level.

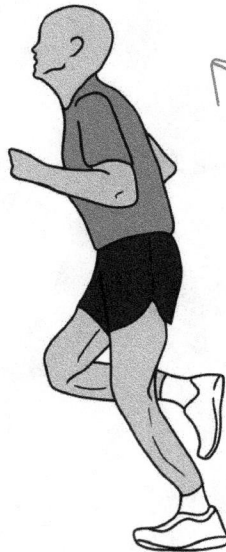

This runner is tilting their head back while leaning forward. We see this a lot when kids try to run faster. You want a tall body and level chin.

THE RUNNING SCHOOL METHOD

Mike Antoniades

Mike invented Dynamic Movement Skills, The Running School Method and Running Re-Education, the method we're going to use to help you improve your running technique and speed.

Mike started The Movement & Running School in 1994, a place where people learn how to run faster, move better, and recover after they've been injured. He's worked with all sorts of people, from kids and everyday runners to super-fast Olympic athletes who've won gold medals! But Mike doesn't just work with athletes. He also helps people who've had strokes or deal with challenges like Parkinson's and MS. His team at The Running School help people move and feel better.

Mike Facts
- Mike has been a coach for more than 40 years and was once a professional football manager and coach.
- He's taught coaches (including me) and health professionals all over the world, including places like the USA, Germany, Norway, Japan, and the Middle East.
- He's featured on podcasts and made videos to help people learn about running, fitness, and even how to stay fit while travelling.
- Mike wrote a book called *Who Taught You How to Run?* aimed at helping adults improve their running technique!

Mike

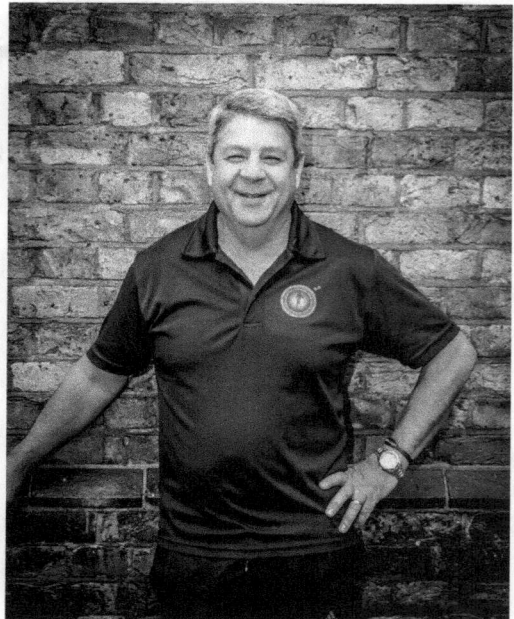

4 Stages of Learning a New Skill

When learning any skill whether school-related or sports-related, there are 4 stages to the learning process. We describe the stages below, but we will do so in relation to running technique;

Unconscious Incompetence (Not Knowing You're Doing It Wrong)
At this stage, you don't realize your running form isn't as good as it could be. You might feel like something is off, or maybe you get tired or hurt, but you're not sure why. It's like you've been doing something the same way for so long, that you don't notice it's not the best way. For example, when runners watch themselves on video, they often say, "I had no idea I was doing that!"

Conscious Incompetence (Knowing What Needs to Change)
Now, you know what's wrong with your running form and what might be causing problems, like getting tired too quickly or getting hurt.
This is the hardest part because fixing it takes a lot of practice and focus. It's especially tough for grown-ups because they've been running the same way for years. For kids, it's usually a bit easier to learn new movements.

Conscious Competence (Getting It Right With Effort)
Your running is much better now, and you can feel the difference! But you still have to think about it while you run. If you're tired or not paying attention, you might slip back into old habits.
With more practice, your body will start to remember the new way of running. It just takes time and effort.

Unconscious Competence (Running Right Without Thinking)
This is when your new running form becomes automatic. You don't have to think about moving your arms or legs a certain way—it just happens naturally! Your brain and body work together to make running feel easy and smooth.

What You Can Expect When Changing Your Technique

Why Does the New Running Technique Feel Hard at First?
When you start learning a new way to run, it might feel harder than the way you usually run. Don't worry – this is totally normal! Here's why it feels tricky in the beginning:

You're trying something new. At first, you'll be focusing a lot on the new technique, and it might feel a bit over the top because you're exaggerating the movements to practice them correctly.

New muscles are working. Your body is using different muscles to push you forward, and these muscles need time to get stronger and used to the new movement.

Your brain is learning, too. Your brain and nerves are working hard to create a new "map" for how your body should move.

But here's the exciting part: After about 4 or 5 weeks, your brain and body will start to adjust. Running will feel smoother, and you'll notice you're spending less time on the ground with each step. That means you're running more efficiently – and faster, too!

How Often Should You Exercise?

Keep Moving!

Exercise and movement, like walking, running, playing, climbing, or jumping, should be part of your daily routine. Kids need to stay active for at least 2 hours every day, and about 45 minutes of that should be more intense, like running around, playing sports, or other activities that get your heart pumping.

Besides what you do at school, it's a great idea to join in running or sports 4-5 times a week.

To make sure your body stays strong and ready to play, it's good to have a balance between exercising and resting. A simple plan is to exercise for 2 days, then rest on the 3rd day to let your body recover and get stronger. I'd recommend at least one rest day per week.

So, lace up your trainers, grab a ball, or head outside, and make movement a fun part of every day!

HOW TO CORRECT YOUR RUNNING TECHNIQUE

Correcting the Leg Cycle

What does an efficient leg cycle look like?

If you watch top athletes run, their legs move in a very specific way:

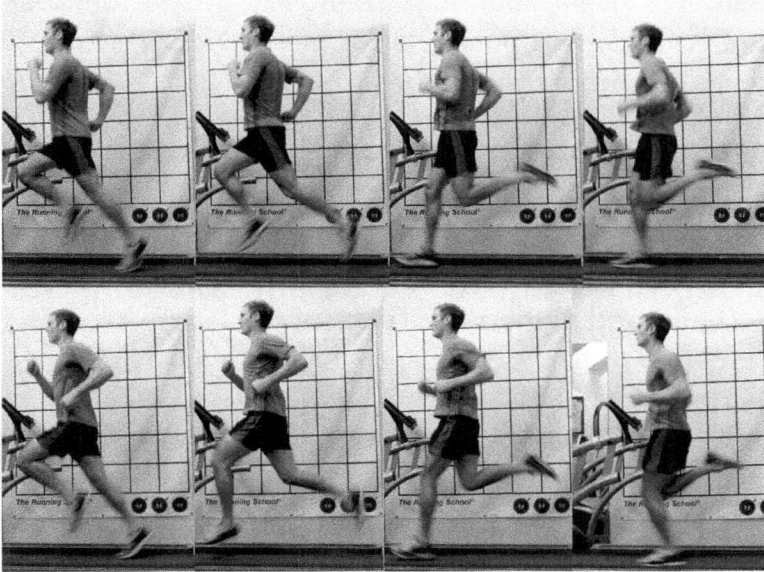

Push Off: When their foot pushes off the ground, their hip stretches back.

Heel Lift: Then, their knee bends, and their heel lifts up high toward their butt.

Swing Through: Next, their leg swings forward in a bent position, making it shorter and easier to move.

Landing: Finally, their feet land just a little in front of their hips, ready for the next step.

This leg movement helps them run fast and efficiently!

This way of running is super efficient because:

No Overstriding: You're not reaching too far forward with your legs, so you don't slow yourself down.

Less Ground Time: Your foot spends less time on the ground because it lands and pushes off closer to your centre of gravity. This gives you more time in the air!

Shorter Leg Movements: Your legs are bent, making them quicker and easier to swing through.

Using Power Muscles: You're using your strongest muscles – your glutes (bum) and hamstrings (back of the legs) – to push forward.

Leg Cycle Practice
Coaching tip: "Cycle Up", "Heels Up"
To practice this, try the leg cycle motion while standing still. This will help you feel what it's like before you do it while running!

1. Stand while holding onto the wall or chair
2. With one leg, extend the leg backwards as if you are scraping gum off your shoe
3. Bend the knee so that the heel comes up toward your bum *(don't kick yourself but almost)*
4. Allow the knee to come forward in front of your body
5. Drop the foot down just ahead of your centre of gravity

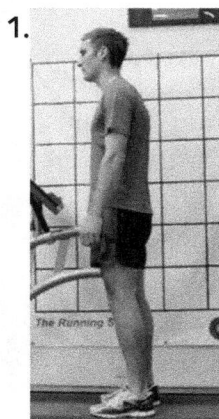

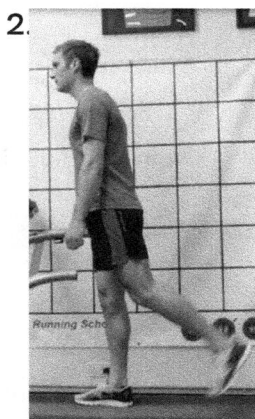

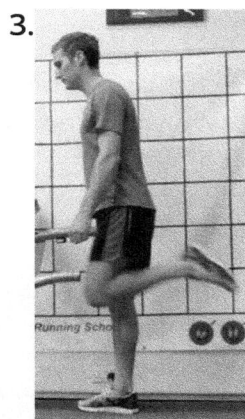

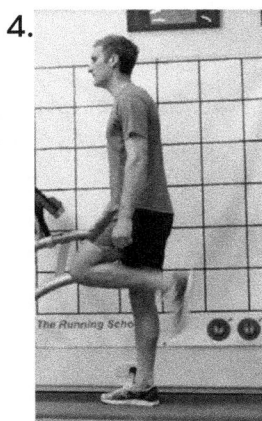

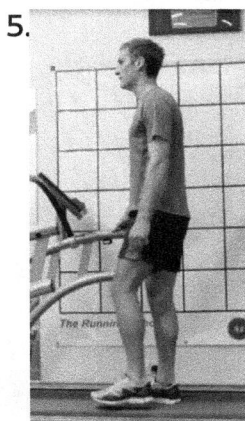

Correcting the Arm Drive

Efficient Arm Drive

Your arms are super important when running! They help you keep your balance, set your rhythm, make you run faster, and even activate your core muscles (the muscles in your tummy and back). The rhythm of your arms also helps your legs move better.

Everyone's arm movement can look a little different because of body shape, flexibility, or how fast they're running. But here are some technique tips to follow:

Bend Your Elbows

Keep your elbows bent at about 90 degrees, like making a letter "L." For long runs, you might feel better bending them a little more – closer to 60 or 45 degrees.

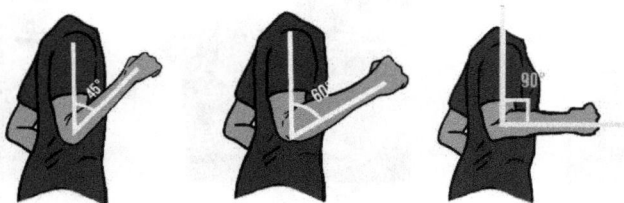

Hold Your Hands Lightly

Pretend you're holding a butterfly in your hands – just enough to keep it safe without squishing it. Put your thumb on top of your fingers, like making a light fist.

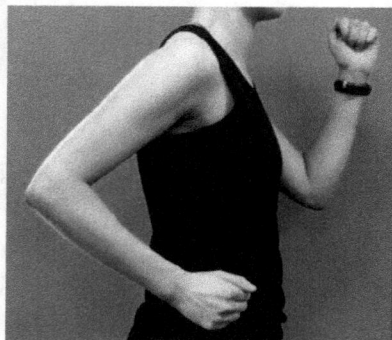

Keep Wrists Facing Your Body

Your wrists should face your body, not the ground. This helps your arms swing forward and backwards properly without twisting your shoulders.

Drive Your Elbows Back

Swing your elbows backward until your hand reaches the top of your hip. This backward movement is super important because it helps push your body forward!

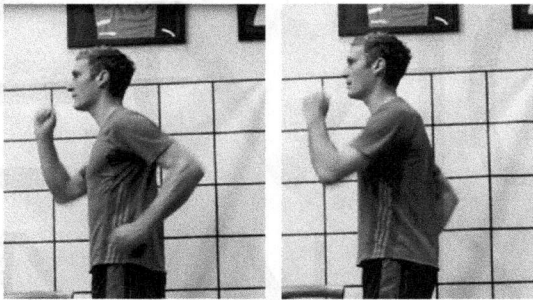

Bring Your Hands Forward

Let your hands come up to just below your chin or shoulder level. How high they go depends on your running speed. But remember: focus on the backward swing, not the forward one – that's what powers your run.

Don't Cross Your Arms

Keep your arms from crossing over the middle of your chest. Crossing them can twist your upper body and throw off how your legs move.

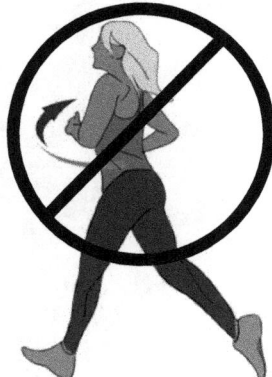

DMS: DYNAMIC MOVEMENT SKILLS

Dynamic Movement Skills

What is DMS and How Does It Work?
DMS (Dynamic Movement Skills) was developed by Mike Antoniades and is all about practising special movements that help your brain and body work better together. These movements stimulate something called the Central Nervous System (CNS), which is like the body's control centre that helps you move properly. By practising these movements over and over again, your brain creates special patterns to help your muscles work more efficiently. This means your body can move faster and better.

Neuromuscular efficiency *(word of the day!)* means your body learns to use the right muscles at the right time to help you move. It also helps your body stay balanced and stable, even when you move in different directions (like running, jumping, or twisting).

What Are the Benefits of DMS?
DMS works your whole body and helps you move in all kinds of ways. Some of the benefits include:

• Better balance and awareness of where your body is in space
• Better coordination for activities like running, jumping, and kicking
• Faster movements and more power (like sprinting or jumping high)
• Improved body control so you don't fall or lose your balance
• More agility to change direction quickly
• A stronger core to help with posture and stability

These improvements start right away after your first practice, and you'll see even bigger changes after about 6 weeks of practice.

Why is It Important to Train Basic Movements?

Basic movement skills are super important because they help kids grow stronger and healthier in their bodies and minds. These skills help you move better, play sports, and even improve how you think and focus in school.

What Are Fundamental Movement Skills?

Fundamental movement skills are the building blocks for doing sports and physical activities. These skills include things like:

- Stability skills (like balancing on one leg)
- Locomotor skills (like running and jumping)
- Manipulative skills (like kicking or throwing a ball)
- These are all the basic moves that help you get better at more complicated sports as you get older.

How Long Does It Take to Learn?

You'll notice some improvements right away after your first practice! But it usually takes about 6 weeks (or 40 days) to really get the hang of the movements and do them smoothly and quickly. That's when you'll start feeling like you can move more easily and with more speed!

Mike teaching me DMS

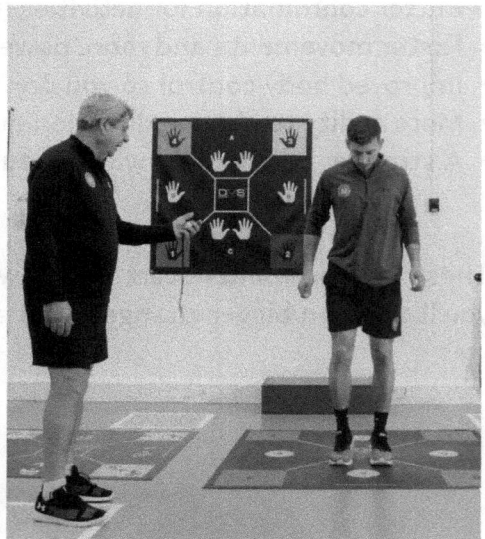

How to plan your DMS Sessions

How to plan your DMS Sessions

The DMS mats can be purchased from our website although you can replicate the DMS Sessions using a large cross on the floor.

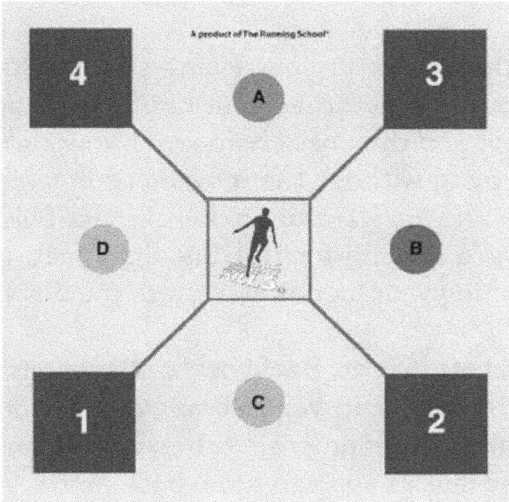

Dynamic Movement Skills Mat.

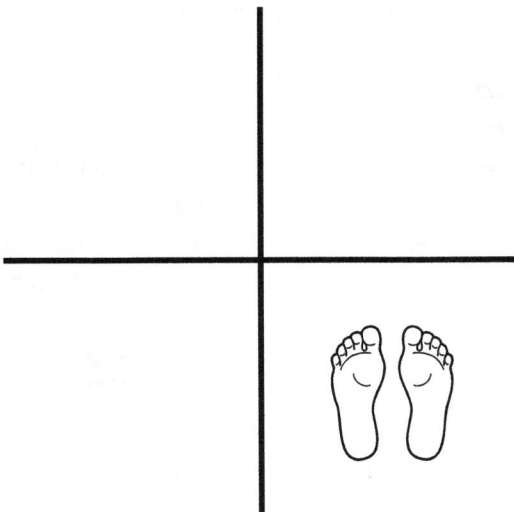

Cross on the floor, ideally a hard floor.

DMS Foundation Movements

Let's take you through the most important DMS movements. You'll use these as part of your warm-up before each running session.

Quick Feet Forwards and Backwards - Left/Right Foot Lead, 20 seconds
Start with both feet behind the line or in your Home square. Step forward across the line with your left foot, then your right. Step back across the line with your left foot and then back home with your right. The goal is to go as fast as you can without the movement breaking down or the wrong foot taking over. You want to do this exercise twice, once for each foot leading. We're looking for fast but light feet, no thumping on the ground or scuffing your feet as this slows you down.

Double Leg Jumps - Forwards, Left, Right, Backwards. 20 seconds
Start with both feet behind the line or in your Home square. Jump forwards (or sideways/backwards depending on the exercise) until your toes cross the line, then as fast as you can jump back home. We want you to jump as fast as you can while staying light on the toes. Try to keep your arms down and no twisting of the feet or body is allowed.

Single Leg Jumps - Forwards, Left, Right, Backwards. 10 seconds
Stand on one leg behind the line or in your Home square. Hop forwards until your toes cross the line, then as fast as you can hop back home. We want you to jump as fast as you can while staying light on the toes. Try to keep your arms down. You'll repeat this exercise so each foot jumps forward, sideways and backwards. Ensure your feet stay straight.

Use a phone camera to scan here to see all the DMS Foundation Movements in action!

RUNNING TECHNIQUE HOMEWORK SESSIONS

How to plan your Running Sessions

The key to practising running technique is to do short bursts of high-quality effort.

Where to hold your running sessions:
These sessions can be carried out at a track, in a park or just a long stretch of grass.

Running Track – everything is painted and set up for you already.
Park, football pitch or green area – Depending on the space you have available you have two options;

Option 1: Lay out three cones/jumpers in a straight line, after the first cone allow a 10-meter gap then a 50-meter gap and then another 10-meter gap.

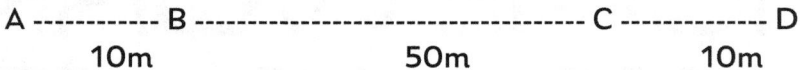

A ------------ B -- C -------------- D
       10m   **50m**   **10m**

Once the cones are laid out the drill is to run from cone A to B and then run at a medium/fast pace concentrating on technique from cones B to C and then jog from C to D. Once completed walk back to Cone A and repeat. This drill should be repeated 10-20 times depending on fitness level.

Option 2: Mark 50-100 metres in a triangle with cones.

What you will need:
•   A watch or stopwatch
•   3/4 x cones
Before starting ensure there are no objects that could cause you to slip, or fall.

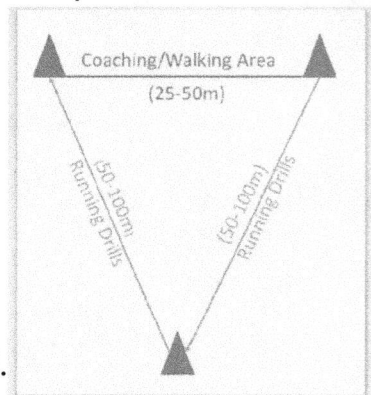

Coaching/Walking Area
(25-50m)

(50-100m) Running Drills

(50-100m) Running Drills

Understanding your Homework

How Often Should I Practice
Each Homework session should be completed two to three times a week. If one of the sessions is very difficult then do it again the following week until it's easy.

Speeds and Paces
In the homework you'll be asked to run at a Slow, Medium and Fast Pace. How can we work that out? The easiest method I find is to use percentages.

100% is going as fast as you can, max speed, cheetah speed and so on.

1% is a very slow walk, think of how a sloth would move (we won't ask you to run at this speed!)

So using the above parameters;
• Slow Pace = 50%
• Medium Pace = 70%
• Fast Pace = 90%

When to Stop the Session
We want quality over quantity when it comes to changing your running technique. Part of our goal is to teach your brain as well as your body, which means that when you're practising your running technique I want it to be as perfect as can be. As soon as you're really tired and can't get your legs up or focus on your technique it's time to head home.

When to Change the Session
This is your homework session, not mine. You may find some of the runs too short or long so feel free to adjust the distance and time so long as you're still focused on that great running technique!

Warming Up with DMS

Do this warm up before each running session.

Dynamic Warmup

1. Dynamic Movement Skills – Quick feet (20 secs, 10 secs rest)
    a.   Leading with the left foot 20 secs Forward
    b.   Leading with the right foot 20 secs Forward
    c.   Leading with the left foot 20 secs Backwards
    d.   Leading with the right foot 20 secs Backwards
    e.   REPEAT SEQUENCE

2.   Jog for 1 minute. Then Walk

3.   Swing, both arms like a windmill, forward gently 10 times and backwards 10 times while you are jogging.

4.   Jog for 2 minutes Then Walk

5.   Dynamic Movement Skills – Quick feet
    a.   Leading with the left foot 20 secs Forward
    b.   Leading with the right foot 20 secs Forward
    c.   Leading with the left foot 20 secs Backwards
    d.   Leading with the right foot 20 secs Backwards

6. Dynamic Movement Skills – Double Leg Jumps (20 secs, 10 secs rest)
    a.   Jumping forwards across a line 20 secs
    b.   Jumping sideways across a line 20 secs Left
    c.   Jumping sideways across a line 20 secs Right
    d.   Jumping backwards across a line 20 secs

7. Let's start running!

Running Technique - Quick Tips

Here's a reminder of our most important changes alongside some coaching cues that I tell our runners, you can have your friend, family member or pet parrot shout these out at you if you slip back into old habits.

Body Position

Try to keep your body tall. Imagine there's a balloon attached to the top of your head lifting you up. *Coaching Cues: "Tall Body", "Chest Up"*

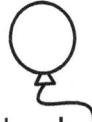

Arm Drive

Imagine you have sweets in your pockets, take a sweet and pop it in your mouth. Pretend sweets only, please! Keep your elbows bent at a right angle. *"Arms Up"*, *"Elbows Back"*, or quite simply *"Arms!"*

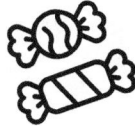

Leg Cycle

Lift your heels towards your bottom, without kicking yourself in the butt! The same way your legs move on a bicycle. This will help you use more muscles and run faster. *"Heels Up", "Legs Up", "Cycle Up"*

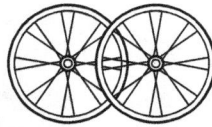

Foot Strike

The fastest way to run is on the balls of the feet. This can take time to learn so it's best to practise in short bursts. If it hurts, then land on your heels until you're ready to try again. *"On the Toes", "Toes"*

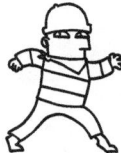

Running Technique—Quick Tips

Here are some of our most important changes. Set aside some reading time ... Occasionally, you can have your friend, family member, or pet parent show these put it, you slip back into old habits.

Body Position

Try to keep your body tall. Imagine there's a balloon attached to the top of your head, lifting you up. Coaching Cues: "Tall Body", "Chest Up".

Arm Drive

Imagine you have swords in your pockets, take a sword and pop it in your mouth. Grab the sweets only, please! Keep your elbows bent at a right angle. "Arms Up", "Elbows Back", or quite simply, "Arms".

Leg Cycle

Lift your heels towards your bottom, without kicking yourself in the butt! The same way you'd use on a move on a bicycle. This will help you use more muscles and run better. "Heels Up", "Legs Up", "Cycle Up".

Foot Strike

The fastest way to run is on the balls of the feet. This can take time to learn, so it's best to practise in short bursts like that, then land on your heel until you're ready to try again. On the ball. "Toes".

SESSION PLANS

Running Technique Homework Session 1

Warm Up 10-15 Minutes

Speed	Sets	Distance/Time	Recovery	Focus
Medium Pace	2	50m or 10secs	Jog Back	Focus on your current running style. Do a couple of runs and pay attention to how you run without applying any of the new coaching tips.
Slow Pace	2	50m or 10secs	Jog Back	Let's start by focusing on the Legs: "Cycle Up". Don't worry about your arms or landing yet.
Medium Pace	5	100m or 20secs	Jog Back	Let's bring the arms in as well! Arm drive: chin to hip. Keep the shoulders relaxed. Sweets in the pockets in to the mouth
Fast Pace	2	50m or 10secs	Jog Back	Let's go faster! Don't forget to use your new technique, even at fast speed!
Medium Pace	8	100m or 20secs	Walk Back	All together now! Arms Up, Cycle Up, Tall Body and Landing on the balls of the feet!
Fast Pace	4	50m or 10secs	Walk Back	Let's speed up! Be careful to maintain your good technique

Running Technique
Homework Session 1

Hey, how did you get on? Feel free to make any notes below with things you found easy, anything you found hard and what you want to focus on more next week.

_____

_____

_____

_____

_____

Nick's Session Notes

This session was all about introducing you to the new technique. It's likely going to feel very strange and quite tiring for the first couple of weeks. That's because we've got new muscles working such as your glutes and hamstrings. We're also concentrating on running like never before, you've got to think about every arm, leg, foot, head position all at one time!

Remember, perfect practice makes permanent! We'll get there together.

Running Technique Homework Session 2

Warm Up 10-15 Minutes

Speed	Sets	Distance/Time	Recovery	Focus
Medium Pace	5	50m or 10secs	Jog Back	Pay attention to how your foot lands. Let's try landing Forefoot and see how it feels. If you're feeling pain then you can switch back to Heel-Toe.
Medium Pace	5	100m or 20secs	Jog Back	Leg Cycle, Arm Drive and Forefoot landing (if pain free).
Medium Pace	2	100m or 20secs	Jog Back	Run 50m with good arm drive then drop your arms and run 50m with hands by your side. Pay attention to what happens. (Arms are important, huh?)
Fast Pace	2	50m or 10secs	Jog Back	Run 25m with good arm drive then start driving the arms really fast for the next 75m. See what happens when you just focus on fast arms!
Medium Pace	8	100m or 20secs	Walk Back	Leg Cycle, Arm Drive and Forefoot landing (if pain free).
Fast Pace	6	50m or 10secs	Walk Back	Let's speed up! Be careful to maintain your good technique

Running Technique
Homework Session 2

Is it starting to feel easier? Feel free to make any notes below with things you found easy, anything you found hard and what you want to focus on more next week.

_____

_____

_____

_____

_____

Nick's Session Notes
I hope the technique is starting to feel more comfortable. In this session, I want to show you how important your arms are to running. Your arm speed will control your leg speed, so next time you want that sudden burst of speed just focus on your arms!

Running Technique Homework Session 3

Warm Up 10-15 Minutes

Speed	Sets	Distance/Time	Recovery	Focus
Medium Pace	5	50m or 10secs	Jog Back	Today's focus is on maintaining your good technique and helping it feel more comfortable. There's going to be lot's of repetition, but remember that's the key to learning a new skill!
MediumPace	6	100m or 20secs	Jog Back	Leg Cycle, Arm Drive and Forefoot landing (if pain free).
Medium Pace	6	100m or 20secs	Jog Back	Leg Cycle, Arm Drive and Forefoot landing (if pain free).
Fast Pace	5	50m or 10secs	Walk Back	Let's go faster! Don't forget - Leg Cycle, Arm Drive and Forefoot landing (if pain free).
Medium Pace	5	100m or 20secs	Walk Back	Leg Cycle, Arm Drive and Forefoot landing (if pain free).
Medium Pace	3	400m or 60secs	Walk Back	Okay let's try some longer runs! Try to keep your good technique for the whole time. If it breaks down that's fine, go back to a walk and finish the rest when you've recovered.

Running Technique Homework Session 3

You made it to week 3! Congratulations, this is the stage that most people give up, remember that learning a new skill is a process! Feel free to make any notes below with things you found easy, anything you found hard and what you want to focus on more next week.

_____

_____

_____

_____

_____

_____

Nick's Session Notes

Technique, technique, technique! Practice, practice, practice! We've added some slightly longer runs into this week's homework.

How does it feel landing on the forefoot, is it feeling faster? Remember it may take you longer to change the way you land so if there's any pain then upi can go back to landing on the heels.

Running Technique Homework Session 4

Warm Up 10-15 Minutes

Speed	Sets	Distance/Time	Recovery	Focus
Medium Pace	5	50m or 10secs	Jog Back	Today's focus is on reinforcing your good technique at faster speeds.
Medium Pace	6	100m or 20secs	Jog Back	Leg Cycle, Arm Drive and Forefoot landing.
Fast Pace	6	75m or 30secs	Jog Back	Let's start going faster! Don't forget - Leg Cycle, Arm Drive and Forefoot landing.
Fast Pace	5	50m or 10secs	Walk Back	Leg Cycle, Arm Drive and Forefoot landing.
Fast Pace	5	100m or 20secs	Walk Back	Leg Cycle, Arm Drive and Forefoot landing.
Max Pace	5	50m or 10secs	Walk Back	Unlock Maximum Speed, Cheetah Speed, 100% Speed!

Running Technique
Homework Session 4

Getting faster! Feel free to make any notes below with things you found easy, anything you found hard and what you want to focus on more next week.

_____

_____

_____

_____

_____

Nick's Session Notes
Of course we're going to try it at 100% speed! How did it feel at your top speed? Did you feel faster?

When we run faster we naturally have less time to think about our technique. That's why it's been important up until now to focus mostly on your Medium Pace, focusing on technique before speed is always the best way. Did it feel more comfortable landing Fore-Foot at the faster speeds?

Running Technique Homework Session 5

Warm Up 10-15 Minutes

Speed	Sets	Distance/Time	Recovery	Focus
Medium Pace	5	50m or 10secs	Jog Back with your old running technique	Today's focus is on not focusing as much!
Medium Pace	5	100m or 20secs	Jog Back with your old technique	Notice the difference between your new running technique and your old technique.
Fast Pace	5	75m or 15secs	Jog Back	Leg Cycle, Arm Drive and Forefoot landing.
Medium Pace	5	50m or 10secs	Jog Back	Do not focus on the technique. Test to see if your technique maintains itself when you are not thinking about it.
Medium Pace	10	100m or 20secs	Walk Back	Do not focus on the technique. Test to see if your technique maintains itself when you are not thinking about it.
Fast Pace	10	50m or 10secs	Walk Back	Leg Cycle, Arm Drive and Forefoot landing.

Running Technique Homework Session 5

We're almost at the end of the course! Feel free to make any notes below with things you found easy, anything you found hard and what you want to focus on more next week.

_____

_____

_____

_____

_____

Nick's Session Notes
After four weeks of paying attention, this week I wanted you to switch off! Has the new technique taken over? Did it feel difficult running with your old style? If so, then we've won! We've successfully changed your technique. If you're still slipping back into the old technique quite easily then that's okay, just more practice is needed.

I've seen some runners change their technique within a week, some over two months. The average is 6-8 weeks.

If it still feels difficult keep trying, it'll soon get much easier!

Running Technique Homework Session 6

Warm Up 10-15 Minutes

Speed	Sets	Distance/Time	Recovery	Focus
Medium Pace	5	100m or 20secs	Jog Back	A great running technique for all speeds. Let's focus on our new technique in the first few runs.
Slow Pace	4	100m or 20secs	Jog Back	Slow it down! Heels cycle up to halfway (about level with the back of your knee), hands come up to your chest.
Medium Pace	4	100m or 20secs	Jog Back	Back to your full Leg Cycle, Arm Drive and Forefoot landing.
Fast Pace	10	100m or 20secs	Walk Back	Leg Cycle, Arm Drive and Forefoot landing.
Max Pace	10	100m or 20secs	Walk Back	Max Speed! Let's Go! Only run again when you've recovered.
Slow/Medium Pace	4	2-3 minutes	Walk Back	Let's try and keep that good technique over a long distance!

Running Technique Homework Session 6

You made it! Feel free to make any notes below with things you found easy, anything you found hard and what you want to focus on moving forward.

_____

_____

_____

_____

Nick's Session Notes

Week 6 is always the most fun. The different speeds make the session a lot more interesting, my apologies for the 2-minute runs!

Why am I practising running slowly? Have you heard the phrase 'life's a marathon, not a sprint'? The same applies to running, sure it would be great if we only ever had to run fast but sometimes you have to slow things down.

Let's take sport for instance. A footballer is on the pitch for 90 minutes but a lot of that time is spent jogging, walking and in my case standing around waiting for someone to pass. Only a small percentage of time is spent sprinting.

When we slow down we want to maintain good technique. So your heels still lift up but just to halfway, about in line with the back of your knee. Your arms still need to drive forward and back but the hands can stop at your chest instead of coming to your chin. When running slowly you may feel more comfortable landing Heel-Toe as well.

Balance

Why is Balance Important for Running?

1. Prevents Wobbling
When you run, you're always moving from one foot to the other. Good balance helps you stay steady so you don't wobble or waste energy.

2. Helps You Run Faster
If your body is balanced, your muscles can focus on pushing you forward instead of correcting your posture. This makes you faster and more efficient.

3. Reduces Injuries
Poor balance can cause uneven movements, which puts extra stress on your feet, ankles, knees, and hips. Good balance helps keep everything aligned and lowers the chance of injuries.

4. Improves Coordination
Balance works with your brain and muscles to keep your movements smooth. This helps your arms and legs work together properly for better running technique.

5. Handles Uneven Surfaces
When you run on trails, grass, or any bumpy surface, balance helps you adapt quickly so you don't trip or fall.

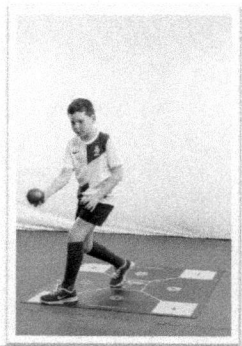

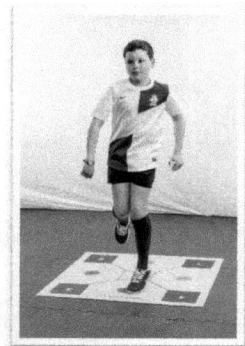

We've designed some balance exercises for you to improve your balance at home!

Single leg balance
Stand on right leg with your left leg in the air behind you, keep the knee soft (slightly bent). Balance for 20-30 seconds. Repeat standing on your left leg. Great to practice when you're brushing your teeth!

Single leg balance with throws and catches
Stand on your right leg with left leg behind you, keep the knee soft. Throw and catch a ball 20 times with a partner or against a wall. Repeat on the left leg. Make it harder by switching arms to catch and throw.

The Famous Running School Balance Game
Well, famous with our runners at least! This one has rules. You vs. a partner.
- Stand about 2 metres away from your partner on one leg.
- You'll need a ball or beanbag.
- Each player starts with 3 lives.
- Your goal is to make your partner lose all their lives.
- To lose a life, you either do a bad throw (too high, wide or uncatchable), you drop the ball, or lose your balance and touch both feet on the ground.
- Start on the left leg, when one of you loses a life you both switch legs.
- You can't lose on the first throw.
- The loser of the first game does five press-ups. The second game is three. Final game is one massive press-up!
- The winner of each round can pick a new ball if you have a few around you.

Conclusion

Running is more than just a sport or exercise—it's a journey of discovery, improvement, and growth. Whether you're learning to run for the first time, or trying to reach a personal best, every step you take is a step toward understanding your body and unlocking its potential.

Throughout this book, we've explored inefficient movement patterns, correct technique, and how with practice you can transform your running. From understanding the importance of balance and arm drive to refining your leg cycle and head posture, every detail contributes to making you a more efficient and confident runner.

Remember These Key Takeaways:

Technique is a Great Word: Small changes, like improving your posture or adjusting your arm drive, can make a big difference.
Consistency Matters: Practice is essential. With repetition, new skills become second nature.
Heels Up, Arms Up, Chest Up: Remember the key coaching points whenever you're running.
Enjoy the Process: Running should be as much about joy as it is about progress. Celebrate your milestones, no matter how small.

As you move forward, take the lessons from this book and make them your own. **Running is a skill, and like any skill, it gets better the more you practice**.

Your journey doesn't end here—it's just the beginning. So lace up your running shoes, get outside, and take the next step. I hope to see you at one of our Running School centres soon and if this book has helped you please let us know.

Your running technique coach and biggest fan,

Nick

Learn With Us

Nick and The Running School have specialised in coaching children aged 6 and up since starting at The Running School.

If you're interested in some one-one coaching at one of our Running School centres you can find your local Running School at www.RunningSchool.com

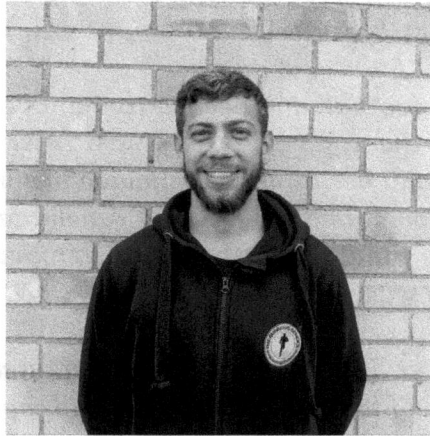

Follow The Running School

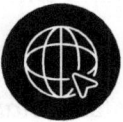 www.RunningSchool.com

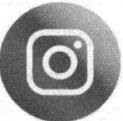 @therunningschool

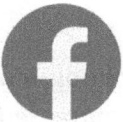 www.facebook.com/runningschoolhq

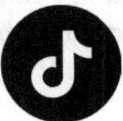 @therunningschool

Praise for The Running School

"*This is our 2nd time using The Running School, Nick and the team are fantastic they go into great detail when analysing my son's running technique. The changes and improvements are nothing short of amazing. I would definitely recommend and I will certainly be using The Running School again. 5 star*" - Dean A

"*My daughter plays football and needed to improve her running speed. We couldn't believe the difference the first 6 sessions has made!! The difference is visible and her running technique has improved massively. Nick is a fabulous coach and really made Amelia feel comfortable and she loved the sessions and found them really enjoyable. She can't wait for her next block to start.*" - Emmie C

"*The guys and girls at The Running School definitely know their stuff. Nick especially is full of first class knowledge and super passionate to get the best out of each individual. After my son's first six sessions his running technique has massively improved, so a massive thank you to all that was involved in making this happen. Look forward to working with you all more in the future, top class!!!!!!*" - Matthew B

"*My son was referred to Nick at The Running School by a professional football academy to make improvements with his acceleration and stride. We booked a 12 week course and the differences are amazing. Nick is very personable and a great coach. Would highly recommend. We will be back for some pre-season sessions. Thanks Nick*" - Jacob and Becci

"*We have had a great experience with Nick at The Running School. My very shy 6 year old has had her confidence boosted and progressed tremendously in the last 6 weeks. Nick is great with children and I can highly recommend the running school. I can't wait to see how much more We can develop our daughter by sending her there.*" - Mandip K

Dot to Dot

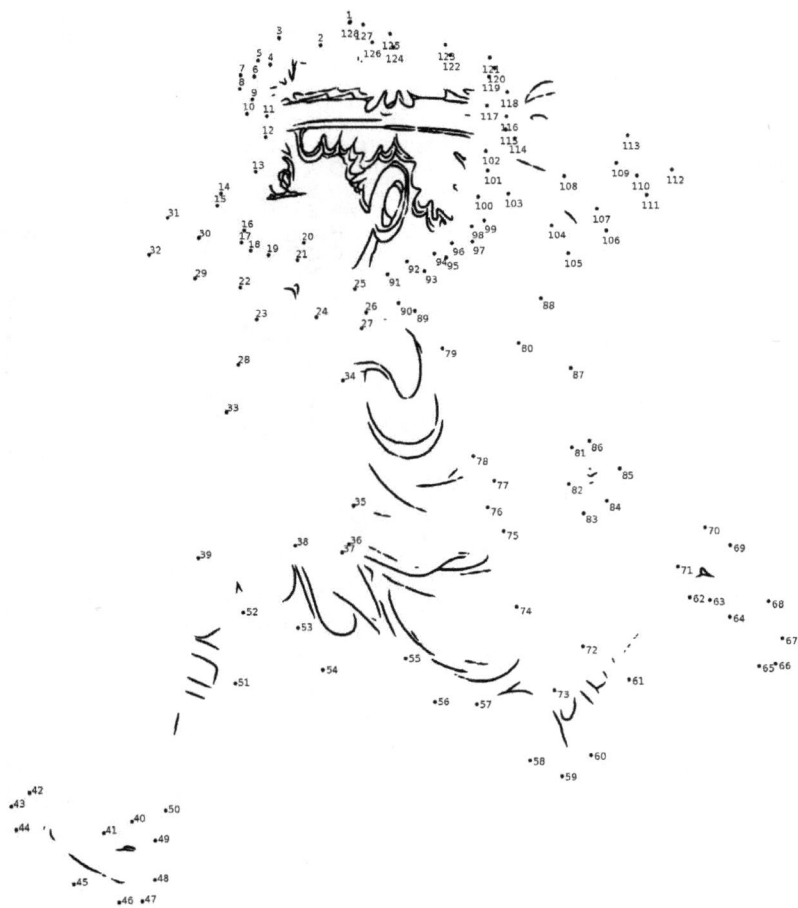

The Running School Word Search

```
Y X C R O S S O V E R T H A W O H W Z C
T V O I B T E Z P J L J T T G T P M C R
C Y X L F I D I M P R O V E E Q V M A P
V O G W A C L X W X U K O W Z I I K J S
X G K R S Z T G T U C O W S B H U X O U
E N A U T W W P H P T U B F C U P R Z C
L P Y N E O X L E H P L H K H C B J B Z
K A G N R C O D R Q N G G C Y C L E M T
L R N I I P O K U J Y C G X S S Z G S H
M I H N F T F Y N A F N M P E P Q W Y N
O T Y G R E R C N V I O W P D A J A T B
V E W P T U T N I L G P A G R M P W F Q
E C D B T A X V N O V E R S T R I D E Z
M H W L B X Y F G M A P F O R E F O O T
E N S A E R X C S Y U A F J X K T X U Q
N I M N P U X O C A V C O S P E E D Y V
T Q J D I N S Y H J A Z W R Z A M M N F
E U P I H N S G O H N U L Q G R F N U K
Y E M N K E C Q O O C H T V O M B M H Y
U O R G B A T A L U M O T S K S W Q E R
```

the running school	technique	crossover	run
overstride	forefoot	movement	
running	improve	landing	
faster	speed	cycle	
arms			

Things I've improved in my running or sport:

_____

_____

_____

_____

Things I've achieved in running or sport since improving my technique:

_____

_____

_____

_____

www.ingramcontent.com/pod-product-compliance
Lightning Source LLC
Chambersburg PA
CBHW060254030426
42335CB00014B/1692